Depression in
General Practice

NEWER INFO
AVAILABLE

This book is to be returned on or before
the last date stamped below.

13 OCT 2003

E06383

Depression in General Practice

André Tylee MD, FRCGP
*RCGP Senior Mental Health Education Fellow
Unit for Mental Health Education in Primary Care
St George's Hospital Medical School
London, UK*

Robert G Priest MD, FRCP (Ed), FRCPsych
Professor of Psychiatry

Ann Roberts BA, MRCPsych, MRCGP
*Research Fellow and
Honorary Senior Registrar
St Mary's Hospital Medical School
London, UK*

MARTIN DUNITZ

© Martin Dunitz Ltd 1996

First published in the United Kingdom
in 1996 by
Martin Dunitz Ltd
The Livery House
7–9 Pratt Street
London NW1 OAE

A CIP record for this book is available from the
British Library.

ISBN 1-85317-288-X

Printed and bound in Spain by Cayfosa

Contents

Introduction   *vii*

Depression   *1*
  What is depression?
  Major depression
  Differential diagnosis
  How common is depression?
  Why does 50% of depression go unacknowledged?
  Patient features
  General practitioner features

The treatment and management of
depression   *14*
  Drug treatment
  Non-drug treatment
  Referral to a psychiatrist

Suicide   *25*
  Risk factors for suicide
  Assessment of suicide risk (general)
  Parasuicide and its relationship to suicide
  Assessment of suicide risk following an attempt
  Prevention of suicide

The skills and training requirements of
general practitioners in mental health today   *38*
  Recognition improves patient outcome
  How to improve recognition
  Questionnaires
  Interviewing skills
  The Unit for Mental Health Education in Primary Care

References   *45*

Index   *53*

Introduction

The aim of this pocketbook is to provide the busy general practitioner and other primary care team members with practical guidance on how to recognize, diagnose and manage depression and suicidal intent.

The book is intended to be practical and reader-friendly and so only essential references are quoted. However, it is hoped that the text has remained as evidence-based as possible.

What is depression?

Whenever a patient mentions the word 'depression' it is important to remember that the word can describe anything from a 'normal' low mood to a life-threatening disorder.[1] A feature common to all depressive conditions is lowering of mood, which, when more severe, may be accompanied by tearfulness and a lack of ability to take interest in or enjoy usual activities. As depression gets worse it becomes more pervasive and a range of other symptoms develop, including negativity, thoughts of personal worthlessness and incapacity, guilt about past actions and pessimism about the future. Thoughts may develop that the person would be better off dead, and these may lead to suicidal intent and action. Sleep and appetite may be either reduced or increased. There may be diurnal mood variation, loss of energy, psychomotor retardation (slowing of movement and speech) or agitation (restlessness, fidgetiness and even pacing up and down) and fears or beliefs of bodily illness. There is often impaired concentration, poor memory or indecisiveness. Anxiety is commonly present, with mixed states being more common than separate ones.

Major depression

Although there is still no universally accepted classification of depression, in practice the criteria are easy to use and it is well worth entering them onto the surgery computer to use as a template.

The essential features of major depression are the presence of depressed mood, or loss of interest and pleasure, together with at least four other symptoms for a minimum duration of 2 weeks, from a list of features described by the DSM-IV criteria (American Psychiatric Association 1994)[2] (Table 1).

Duration of at least two weeks	
One of either:	depressed mood *or*
	markedly diminished interest or pleasure in normal activities
Plus four of:	significant weight loss or gain
	insomnia or hypersomnia
	agitation or retardation
	fatigue or loss of energy
	feelings of worthlessness or excessive guilt
	reduced ability to concentrate or make decisions
	thoughts of death or suicidal thoughts or actions

Table 1
Diagnostic criteria for major depression (American Psychiatric Association 1994)[2]

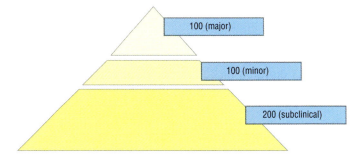

Figure 1
Incidence of depression on an average GP's list of 2000 patients

The general practitioner (GP) with an average list size of around 2000 patients may have up to 100 patients with major depression at any one time and another 100 patients with milder depression (i.e. presenting with only two or three of the criteria from the list in Table 1, rather than four) (Figure 1).

Several of these people with milder depression will have chronic mild fluctuating depression (dysthymia). Dysthymia is a chronic disturbance involving either depressed mood or loss of interest or pleasure in all or most usual activities which is not of a severity or duration to meet the definition for major depression, but which must have been present for 2 years or more with no more than a few months free from symptoms. In addition to the low mood, at least two of the following must be present:

- Poor or increased appetite
- Poor or increased sleep
- Low energy
- Low self-esteem
- Poor concentration
- Feelings of hopelessness

There are also up to 200 people at any one time on a GP's list who may have 'subclinical' depression (i.e. below the level of milder depression or dysthymia).

Manic-depressive disorder (bipolar illness) is characterized by periods of elevated mood in addition to depression, which when present tends to be more severe and recurrent. On average, a typical GP's list will feature less than 10 patients in this category.

The tenth revision of the International Classification of Diseases (ICD-10)[3] provides a slightly different classification of depressive illness: it describes depressive episodes as mild, moderate or severe, depending on the number of symptoms and severity (Table 2).

Both the systems described above for diagnosing depression are useful and either can be chosen for everyday use.

Differential diagnosis

In a general practice setting it is important to remember that the diagnosis of major depression may be secondary to organic factors. Organic factors include drugs (corticosteroids, diuretics, reserpine, methyldopa, barbiturates), endocrine conditions (hypothyroidism, Cushing's syndrome, Addison's disease), infections (influenza, hepatitis, glandular fever, brucellosis, herpes zoster), malignancies (carcinomas of the pancreas, lung or brain), brain disorders (cerebrovascular accidents, multiple sclerosis, Parkinson's disease, epilepsy, dementia), kidney disease (renal failure, dialysis), haematological disorder (iron deficiency anaemia, folate deficiency, vitamin B_{12} deficiency) and drug withdrawal (benzodiazepines, amphetamines, alcohol).

If the patient presents with a low mood, ask:

1 How bad is it and how long has it been going on?
2 Have you lost interest in things?
3 Are you more tired than usual?

If the answer is 'yes' to any of the above, continue:

4 Have you lost confidence in yourself?
5 Do you feel guilty about things?
6 Do you find it difficult to concentrate?
7 How are you sleeping?
8 Have you lost your appetite/any weight?
9 Do you feel that life is not worth living any more?

How severe is the depression?

Mild
At least two criteria from 1–3, plus two others.

Moderate
At least two criteria from 1–3, plus three or four others and/or 'yes' to question 5.

Severe
Most of the criteria listed above in severe form and/or 'yes' to questions 5 and 9.

Table 2
ICD-10 criteria for depression (modified for the Defeat Depression Campaign by Armstrong and Lloyd[4])

Second, depression is unacknowledged because GPs may differ in their characteristics or consulting behaviour (Table 4).

Increasing recognition	Knowledge:
	about the symptoms of depression
	about the treatments available
	Attitudes:
	showing interest and concern
	asking about the home, work and family
	sensitivity to verbal and non-verbal cues
	Skills in interviewing:
	giving eye-contact
	listening
	asking open-ended questions initially
	asking about feelings
	making empathetic comments
	asking directive questions when appropriate
Decreasing recognition	Conservative personality types
	A tendency to prescribe hypnotics
	A tendency to ask irrelevant questions
	A tendency to ask closed questions

Table 4
Doctor features that affect the recognition of depression

Patient features

Marks and colleagues[13] found that male patients are more likely to have their psychiatric health rated accurately by their doctor, and that GPs were most accurate with middle-aged patients. Widowed patients and female patients were more likely to be perceived as psychiatrically disturbed. Patients aged 15–24, the unemployed and students were least likely to have their psychiatric illness recognized.

Most contacts with GPs are initiated by patients, and differences in their help-seeking behaviour will affect the consultation. A general population survey[14] commissioned for the launch in 1992 of the UK Defeat Depression Campaign organized by the Royal College of Psychiatrists in association with the Royal College of General Practitioners found that most people felt that depression carried a stigma and that their GPs might consider them lacking in 'backbone' or be unsympathetic. Many respondents wanted to be listened to but thought that their GP did not have enough time. They did not want antidepressant pills because they (mistakenly) thought them to be addictive. A more recent survey indicates an improvement in this last misconception.[15]

Those patients who do discuss their depressive symptoms are more likely to complain of hopelessness, cognitive difficulties, loss of appetite and loss of weight.[16] Such patients are typically aged over 36, have bad physical health, and will have used mental health facilities before. They are female, recently separated or widowed and also have got panic and phobic disorders. Patients who abuse drugs or are drug-dependent are less likely to discuss depressive symptoms.[17]

A key task for the GP is to distinguish between psychiatric and non-psychiatric disorder and then between forms of psychiatric disorder. Two symptoms may be valuable in pointing to depression: depressed mood which is persistent and pervasive; and loss of motivation, interest and drive.[18] These two symptoms can be used as screening questions when depression is suspected.

Those patients whose depression goes unacknowledged look less depressed, are less likely to attribute their illness to depression, are more likely to have had their depressive illness for over a year and typically have a physical illness.[7]

Such patients are more likely to be somatizing their distress by seeking help from the GP for the somatic symptoms of their psychiatric disturbance.[8] Somatization may account for half of all undetected psychiatric disorder, whilst nearly half of the remaining unrecognized group may have a physical illness. A somatizer is often difficult to convince of the need for psychiatric treatment.[19]

It is interesting to note that psychiatrists assessing patients in a general practice setting had difficulty judging whether the patients had a discrete psychiatric diagnosis when physical illness was present,[20] indicating just how difficult it often is to make holistic or multiaxial diagnoses in the primary care setting.

Patients who are more depressed are more likely to give cues (verbal, vocal and postural) in their consultations, but some doctors seem to suppress the expression of verbal and vocal (but not postural) cues by their patients.[21]

Patients whose depression is more likely to be recognized are those who present with a psychological or social reason; those who present symptoms of more recent origin; and those with more than one psychiatric diagnosis and severe illness.

Also, patients who have received a psychiatric diagnosis from their GP in the previous year are more likely to be recognized at re-presentation than those presenting for the first time.[22,23]

Female patients with physical illness seen by GPs are up to five times less likely to have a concurrent major depression recognized than female attenders who have no physical illness at all.[24] Women with mild physical illness and major depression are nearly three times less likely to have the depression recognized than women who have major depression alone.

The content of a consultation differs in consultations that lead to recognition in that women who mention a psychological symptom early are more likely to have their depression recognized.[25]

General practitioner features

A doctor's failure to acknowledge depression might arise from any of the following:[26]

- A lack of knowledge regarding depressive symptoms and their management

- A failure to consider the diagnosis of depression because of a preoccupation with possible organic pathology

- A failure to elicit affective, cognitive, and/or somatic symptoms relevant to the diagnosis of depression

- An under-rating of depression's severity or treatability after considering this diagnosis relative to the competing medical ones

- An awareness of the presence of depression, but a failure to diagnose it because psychiatric illness is not properly treated in primary care practice

General practitioners' knowledge

'Age and experience' (years in practice, age and higher qualifications) do not show strong associations with accuracy.[13] Academically more able doctors who possess an appropriate concept of minor psychiatric illness are more likely to rate their patients' degree of emotional distress accurately and use more directive interview approaches.

General practitioners' skills

General practitioners who are more accurate than others in recognizing depression[27] tend to make more eye-contact with the patient, to be less likely to interrupt the patient or show signs of being in a hurry, and to be 'good listeners'. They are also more likely to ask direct questions with a psychological and social content. Doctors who inhibit a depressed patient ask many 'closed' questions (questions readily answered by 'yes' or 'no') and questions derived from theory rather than what the patient has said.

Doctors able to detect psychiatric illness are more likely to allow patients to express verbal cues about mood and permit 'vocal' (para-verbal) cues such as sighing.[21]

General practitioners' attitudes

General practitioners can be classified as faster (average of 6.99 minutes or less per patient), intermediate and slower (9.0 minutes or more per patient) in their length of consultation, and patient satisfaction is greater with longer consultations, which are more likely to include psychosocial problems.[28]

When a GP shows 'interest and concern' and empathy,[29] is interested in psychiatry and asks questions about family, they are more likely to correctly recognize depression.[13] However, 'conservative' doctors who resist change tend to be extraverts, prescribe hypnotics, make irrelevant statements during consultations and miss depression.[13]

A first step to improving recognition is to know the range of depressive symptoms to ask about, and one way of doing this is to keep an *aide memoire* on paper or perhaps as a template on a computer, as is often done for other conditions such as diabetes.

Whilst concern about physical illness is desirable, it is not appropriate for all patients to be investigated for organic disorder before the psychosocial aspects of their problems are tackled.

For the GP, the main conclusion is the importance of familiarity with a relatively direct interview for the specific symptoms of depression and of being willing to ask these questions in a sensitive and empathetic way.

Summary

Depression is a common condition and is eminently treatable if recognized. A combined approach that encourages patients to discuss it more readily and GPs to be more willing and able to manage it with the help of the primary health care team seems at present to be the most pragmatic approach. Ways of improving the recognition of depression are discussed further in the final chapter (page 38).

The treatment and management of depression

The key to effective management is recognition of the depression itself. Because of concern in the UK that about half of those persons in the community suffering from serious degrees of depression do not approach their doctors for treatment, and that the GPs themselves recognize only about half of those that do present, the Royal College of Psychiatrists in association with the Royal College of General Practitioners launched the Defeat Depression Campaign in 1992.[30] This aimed at educating the public in the treatable nature of depressive illness and at improving the knowledge of health care professionals in both the recognition and the treatment of depression. The scientific basis of the campaign was established by a joint consensus meeting.[31]

There have been similar campaigns in the USA and in Ireland, but the most striking short-term results of such an educational programme in general practice were found in the Swedish island of Gotland.[32]

General practitioners on this island were given an intensive course on the recognition and treatment of depression. Immediately following this exercise, there were profound falls in the rates of admission to hospital for depressive illness and in the incidence of suicide (particularly in females). Sick leave for depression was reduced. Prescriptions of antidepressants and lithium increased, and prescriptions for anxiolytics and hypnotics fell.[33] Unfortunately, within a short period of time the benefits of this programme were lost. There is clearly a need for follow-up activity to reinforce such exercises.

The UK Defeat Depression Campaign has gone some way to address this issue and it makes recommendations for the appropriate treatment of the condition.[31] Management of depressive illness usually involves a combination of treatment modalities and it is not uncommon to combine pharmacological and psychotherapeutic approaches. The patient's wishes must be borne in mind when deciding on a treatment programme, as otherwise compliance will be poor.

Drug treatment

This usually involves the prescribing of an antidepressant, although other drugs may sometimes be given in combination. Antidepressants are highly effective in the treatment of depressive disorders which satisfy the criteria for major depressive episodes lasting more than 2 weeks. They have greatest efficacy in episodes which are moderate or severe, and they take about two weeks to start having an effect. Antidepressants should not be withheld just because the depression seems understandable, but should be offered to all patients who meet the criteria, irrespective of cause. As well as treating the acute phase of the illness, it is also necessary to give antidepressants throughout the continuation phase and in some cases to provide prophylaxis (Figure 2). Evidence for this comes from a few well-controlled long-term treatment studies.[34–38] Most of this evidence, as for most information regarding the treatment of depression, has been derived from hospital outpatients and this may not reflect the true picture in general practice.

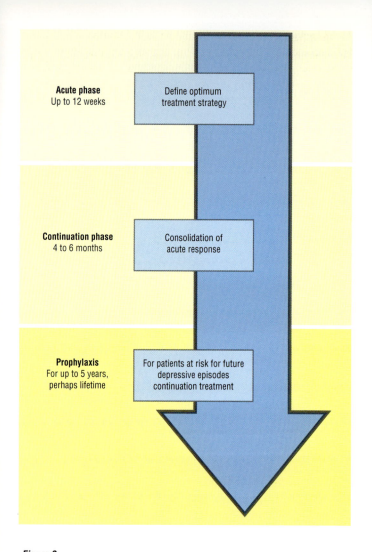

Acute phase
Up to 12 weeks

Define optimum
treatment strategy

Continuation phase
4 to 6 months

Consolidation of
acute response

Prophylaxis
For up to 5 years,
perhaps lifetime

For patients at risk for future
depressive episodes
continuation treatment

Figure 2
Treatment phases in depression. (Reproduced with the kind premission of Dr J.
G. C. Rasmussen.)

Acute-phase treatment

This phase relates to the length of time it takes for the medication to enable the patient to feel normal. The precise length of this period varies and is dependent on many factors, such as compliance, severity of illness and dose of medication. Usually this takes about eight weeks but it may take much longer and treatment must be continued until remission is achieved.

Continuation-phase treatment

This relates to the time needed to consolidate the initial response to the antidepressant and prevent relapse. It requires treatment with the same drug as used in the acute phase of therapy, at the *same dose* for a further 4–6 months. If patients fail to continue with their antidepressants for this additional period, there is a 50% chance of deterioration within the following 6 months (compared with 20% when treatment is continued). Patients need to be encouraged to take their medication throughout this period and warned of the risks of stopping it prematurely. This policy should be pursued even in first episodes of depressive illness in primary care.

Prophylaxis

This refers to the prevention of further episodes of depression by continuing with medication, possibly indefinitely. Prophylaxis should be considered when there have been severe recurrent episodes of illness. To date, the optimal length of prophylactic treatment with antidepressants is unclear. The dose of antidepressants during this phase of treatment is not well established, but long-term treatment studies show that doses are likely to be similar to those used in acute treatment. The decision regarding prophylaxis should be a joint one with the patient, and the benefits must be balanced against the risks. Some psychiatrists now advocate lifelong treatment with antidepressants for those who are most vulnerable.

Tricyclic antidepressants (TCAs)

Most GPs continue to use these drugs as first-line treatment of depression because of familiarity with them and cost. Although most efficacy data come from hospital studies, there is evidence that TCAs work in the acute phase of depressive illness in general practice populations.[39-42] The dose of TCAs is important if a response is to be achieved. In general practice, doses of 125–150 mg daily are effective in treating depression.[39,42] Lower doses are not effective.[43] In the case of lofepramine, the effective dose is 210 mg daily. Insufficient doses are frequently prescribed in general practice, thereby reducing the chance of recovery.

Side-effects of TCAs

TCAs can cause a variety of adverse effects:

- Anticholinergic side-effects, such as dry mouth, constipation, urinary problems and visual problems; these are all commoner in the elderly
- Drowsiness
- Weight gain
- Sexual problems
- Confusion (especially in the elderly)
- Cardiac arrhythmias (especially in overdose)

TCAs are particularly dangerous in overdose. Since 15% of patients with major depression commit suicide, the risk of overdose needs to be considered in all depressed patients and not just in those who admit to suicidal thoughts or those with previous suicide attempts.

Selective serotonin reuptake inhibitors (SSRIs)

These drugs are as effective as the TCAs in the first-line treatment of the acute phase of depressive illness and are effective in preventing recurrent episodes.[44] Overall they are better tolerated than TCAs and this should lead to better compliance, which is important in view of the frequency with which TCAs are abandoned by patients prematurely. The SSRIs are more likely to be taken in adequate daily amounts, whereas the TCAs are often taken at sub-therapeutic dosage. They have other important advantages. Firstly, they are not toxic in overdose and this is a major advantage over earlier treatments. Secondly, they produce less psychomotor retardation when compared with the TCAs.[45] This is increasingly becoming an important issue, particularly in relation to road traffic accidents.

Side-effects of SSRIs

The side-effects commonly associated with SSRIs are:

- Nausea and other gastrointestinal problems
- Sweating
- Headache
- Sexual problems

Most of these side-effects disappear within 2 weeks of treatment, unlike side-effects of the TCAs. As with other serotonergic drugs, the rare complication of the serotonin syndrome may occur, in which muscular overactivity (restlessness, tremor, myoclonus and so on) leads to hyperpyrexia. This must be treated as an emergency, e.g. with curarization and mechanical ventilation.

The SSRIs are particularly useful in treating depression with associated obsessional symptoms or bulimia. They have been widely studied in prophylactic treatment in mixed hospital and general practice populations. There is good evidence that they are effective in preventing recurrent episodes.

Other antidepressants

Of the newer classes of antidepressant, the reversible inhibitors of monoamine oxidase (RIMA), e.g. moclobemide, do not possess the risk of 'cheese reactions' seen with the older monoamine oxidase inhibitors (MAOIs). Their side-effect profile is benign and they do not appear to be toxic in overdose. The classical MAOIs still have a place in the treatment of depression, particularly in those patients with milder illness associated with high anxiety levels or panic attacks, but their use is limited in general practice because of their serious interactions with certain foods and other drugs.

One recent introduction, venlafaxine, is active on both the serotonergic and noradrenergic neurotransmitter systems. In contrast to the TCAs, it has no significant effect on the muscarinic, histaminergic or other neurotransmitter systems. The usual treatment dose is 75–150 mg daily in divided doses,although higher doses (up to 375 mg daily) can be used where clinically indicated. Other drugs such as mianserin and trazodone occasionally have a place in the treatment of some patients.

The use of other drugs in depression

Antipsychotic drugs have a place in the treatment of psychotic depression although many of these patients show a good response to electroconvulsive therapy (ECT). Thioridazine in small doses is often useful in controlling severe anxiety. Benzodiazepines have only a minor role to play. They may be considered in patients with severe sleep disturbance or anxiety. If prescribed they should be used on an intermittent basis and for no longer than 2 weeks continuously. Lithium is particularly

useful in the treatment of resistant depression and in the prophylaxis of bipolar affective disorder, and GPs may be involved
with the blood level monitoring of this drug.

Drug treatment of depression can be readily combined with
psychological treatment and should be in many patients. A programme of treatment should be negotiated with the patient,
whose wishes can thereby be taken into account.

Non-drug treatment

Counselling and more specific therapies may be useful for
patients with milder forms of the illness and for those with a
chronic course who are not severely ill at presentation.
Studies have been undertaken in both the acute phase of a
depressive illness and in the longer term. There have also
been studies comparing the outcome of patients treated with
antidepressants alone, psychotherapy alone, and a combination of the two. Evidence is growing for the belief that
certain psychological treatments can reduce the risk of
recurrent episodes of depression, whether used only in the
acute phase or continued beyond remission for a defined
period. In order to engage in psychological treatments
patients cannot be too ill, since in severe depression thinking processes are slowed and distorted, impeding the
patient's ability to respond to a 'talking' approach. They may
have to be treated initially with antidepressants and continue with them in order to remain well enough to engage in
therapy.

Cognitive behaviour therapy
This therapy rests on the premise that the patient's depression
results directly from a negative view of himself or herself and
the surrounding world.[46] The therapy attempts to bring about
improvement in depressive symptoms by challenging the
patient's negative assumptions. Typically it is conducted by

clinical psychologists. Blackburn[47] compared cognitive therapy, antidepressant medication, and a combination of the two in both a hospital and a general practice setting. Subjects who had initially responded to a 12–15-week treatment course were assigned to ongoing therapy for a further 6 months. At the end of this period there was no significant difference in level of illness in any of the groups. After a further 18 months without treatment, patients were reassessed for relapse and recurrence of depressive illness. In the medication-only group, 78% had deteriorated, whereas only 23% of the cognitive-therapy-alone group and 21% of the combination group suffered a relapse or recurrence.

Interpersonal therapy

This was initially developed as a supportive measure for depressed patients.[48] It aims toward symptomatic relief, through addressing conflicts or deficits in the patient's social sphere. The most convincing evidence for efficacy of this therapy in the short-term management of depression comes from a comparative study in the USA.[49, 50] Patients received 16 weeks' treatment with interpersonal therapy, pharmacotherapy, a combination of both or non-scheduled supportive therapy on demand. After this initial treatment period, all three active treatments performed comparably and significantly better than the non-scheduled treatment.

Patients were reassessed after a year and no group differences were found in the level of illness or in the frequency of relapse. Another study by Elkin[51] compared 16 weeks of treatment with imipramine, cognitive therapy, interpersonal therapy or drug placebo. At the end of treatment, outcome was best in the imipramine group and worst in the placebo group, with the two psychotherapies in between. Follow-up assessments were conducted at 6, 12 and 18 months after termination of therapy and survival analyses revealed no significant differences between all four groups.

Clearly, although these therapies are efficacious they cannot easily be fitted into a general practice setting. They require considerable time and training on the part of the therapist, whether a physician or another health professional. The initial cost of such therapies is more than the cost of prescribing an antidepressant, since a course of treatment usually takes at least 12 one-hour sessions; but they may prove more cost-effective in the long run by preventing future episodes or illness. More studies need to be done to establish the health economics of such treatment.

Other psychological treatments

Some studies in general practice have shown that counselling is helpful in specific settings. Depressed patients with marital problems have been treated by social workers[52,53] and women with non-psychotic postnatal depression have responded to treatment by health visitors given minimal training in Rogerian counselling.[54] A recent study failed to reveal any difference in efficacy between a problem-solving approach and 150 mg daily of amitriptyline in the short-term treatment of mild depression, suggesting that either is effective.[42]

Referral to a psychiatrist

Not all depressive illness can be treated in the community. Some is too severe and requires hospital admission, particularly if the patient is a high suicide risk or is no longer eating or drinking. The GP may require the services of a psychiatrist in an outpatient setting. This is particularly useful if there is doubt about the diagnosis, or if the patient has a dual diagnosis, such as the addition of alcoholism or obsessive–compulsive disorder. Sometimes patients are resistant to treatment and the GP may request the advice of a psychiatrist for further management. If there is an issue about prophylactic treatment, the GP may wish the patient to be seen by a psychiatrist for a second opinion. Depressed patients sometimes become angry with their GP, believing them to be inexperienced in the management of their illness. They may request to see a specialist, but often when this happens the psychiatrist does nothing different from the GP. The patient's anger may be a sign of the frustration felt when relief from the symptoms of depression takes a long time. In some areas, referral to a psychiatrist is the only route to more specialized services, such as community psychiatric nurses (CPNs), social workers and clinical psychologists. Some general practices have circumvented this problem by employing their own CPNs and other clinical specialists. There should be easily accessible liaison between the GP and the local psychiatrist to prevent the GP feeling completely isolated in the management of this often difficult disorder. This may be facilitated by regular visits by a psychiatrist to the surgery. It is by cooperation amongst different professionals that the patients receive the optimal treatment for their depressive illness.

Suicide

The frequency of suicide has a significant impact on society. The incidence varies between countries, with the highest being in Hungary (4.5 per 10 000) and the lowest in Egypt and Jamaica (0.01 per 10 000, see Table 5). It may not be possible to directly compare these rates, since countries vary in the methods used to derive these figures.

Country	Suicide rates per 10 000 population (WHO statistics 1988)
Hungary	4.53
Denmark	2.78
France	2.27
USA	1.23
England & Wales	0.89
Italy	0.78
Argentina	0.63
Philippines	0.05
Jamaica, Egypt	0.01

Table 5
International suicide rates

Since suicide affects young people, it contributes to life years lost amongst the general population and has both economic and social consequences. For these reasons, in the UK, suicide reduction is a target in the *Health of the Nation* document published by the Secretary of State for Health in 1992.[55,56] The targets are to reduce the overall suicide rate by at least 15% and to reduce the suicide rate amongst severely mentally ill people by at least 33%, both by the year 2000. This is indeed a challenge, since it is not clear from current research whether or not suicide is always preventable or whether any reduction in the suicide rate can be maintained over time.

General practitioners are only rarely exposed to cases of suicide, with the average GP seeing one every 4–5 years. However, 40% of people who commit suicide have had contact with their GP during the previous month and about 20% have seen their GP during the week prior to death.[57,58] This suggests that perhaps GPs are ideally positioned to have an impact on the reduction of the suicide rate but in fact these figures mean only that the average GP will see someone shortly before that person commits suicide once every 8–10 years. Nevertheless, the study in Sweden[33] has shown that where GPs become skilled at recognizing and treating depression effectively, the suicide rate can fall dramatically.

Suicide statistics are based on the verdicts returned at inquests. These verdicts do not necessarily reflect the true suicide rate, since such a verdict can be reached only if there is sufficient evidence that the death was self-inflicted *and* that the person intended to end his or her life. If this cannot be proved, an open verdict is returned. It has been suggested that suicide statistics would be more accurate if the civil, rather than the criminal, standard of proof could be applied during inquests.[59]

Risk factors for suicide

There are many such factors but this does not mean that suicide is always predictable or preventable. Risk factors only act as guidelines in the overall assessment of the patient. Table 6 shows the main risk factors for completed suicide.

Older males

Isolation (divorced, widowed, single)

Recently bereaved

Psychiatric illness (especially affective disorders and alcoholism)

Past attempt (extremely important; see below)

Unemployment

Physical illness (especially in the elderly)

Table 6
Risk factors for suicide

Men have traditionally had a higher suicide rate than women but there have recently been changes in the age-related suicide rate amongst men. Until the 1960s the male rate gradually increased with age, but currently in the UK there is a peak of male suicides amongst the 15–25-year age group as well as the increase in old age. The reasons for this are unclear, but high unemployment rates with a sense of hopelessness may be important. Men tend to use more violent methods of suicide than women, who more often take drug overdoses.

Psychiatric illness is an extremely important risk factor for suicide. There have been a number of large retrospective studies of completed suicides.[60–64] The overall findings of these studies are that virtually all were thought to have suffered from a psychiatric disorder – approximately 50% affective disorder, 25% alcoholism, 5% schizophrenia, and 20% other disorders, such as personality disorder or neurosis.

In the study of elderly suicides[64] 65% had a physical illness. At least 50% of people who commit suicide have had contact with psychiatric services in the past and 25% are in contact at the time of their death. Psychiatric patients who have recently been discharged from inpatient care are particularly at risk. It is often during the recovery phase of illness that suicide risk is greatest, although this is not true for depression. Table 7 shows the life-time risk of suicide for each major psychiatric disorder.

Affective disorder	15%
Alcoholism	15%
Schizophrenia	10%
Personality disorder	10%

Table 7
Life-time risk of suicide for major psychiatric disorders

Patients with depression who kill themselves often have marked symptoms of hopelessness, guilt, insomnia or impaired memory. Psychomotor retardation does not necessarily protect against suicide, with 50% of suicide completers having this feature. Alcoholism is associated with a high mortality rate, both because of the high morbidity from physical complications and because 15% of alcoholics eventually commit suicide.

Unlike with affective disorders, this occurs at a late stage in the course of the illness. The majority are depressed because alcohol, in the long term, acts as a depressant on mood, but other related risk factors include poor physical health, poor employment record, past history of suicidal behaviour and recent loss of a close relationship.

Schizophrenia is associated with a 10% life-time risk of suicide. It is more likely in the early stages of the illness, often when the individual has regained insight after a period of hospitalization. Young men seem particularly at risk but this may just reflect the fact that schizophrenia presents at an earlier age in men than in women. Those who had achieved a high level of educational status prior to the onset of the illness are more likely to commit suicide, as are those who are unemployed. The extrapyramidal side-effect of neuroleptics known as akathisia (pathological restlessness) and abrupt withdrawal of medication make patients particularly vulnerable, and most have expressed ideas of hopelessness or a fear of mental disintegration prior to killing themselves.

The risk of suicide in people with a diagnosis of neurosis varies according to the types of symptom. Patients with panic disorder or with mild depression are particularly at risk, whereas those with obsessive–compulsive disorder have a low rate of suicide. Some personality problems also predispose to suicide and people most at risk are those with lability of mood, aggression, poor impulse control, feelings of alienation from peers and associated drug or alcohol problems. The effect of unemployment on suicide risk is complicated. Although it is common in suicide completers, it is not clear whether it is a primary cause or a consequence of some other factor such as psychiatric disorder.

For the GP, the two most important predictors of suicide are:

- Current thoughts of suicide
- Recent suicide attempt (even if apparently trivial)

Both of these factors are associated with a risk of suicide in the following year, approximately *100 times that of the general population*.

These factors will now be considered further.

Assessment of suicide risk (general)

This has been studied in depth by Hawton.[65] For any patient it is important to establish whether or not suicidal thoughts are present, especially if the individual suffers from a psychiatric disorder. It is not always easy to ask about such thoughts if the patient has not expressed them spontaneously. Most patients welcome the opportunity to talk about their ideas. If they are not given this chance, they may go away feeling misunderstood and isolated, thereby increasing the risk of suicide in those who harbour such thoughts. Doctors must learn by practising how to feel comfortable when asking about suicidal ideation. Often it helps to explore a patient's thinking by asking graded questions: quite general questions at first, followed by more direct ones. This can be achieved only if the doctor has established good rapport with the patient.

Examples of general questions are:

- Do you ever think that life is not worth living?
- Do you ever wish that you would not wake up in the morning?
- Do you sometimes wish that your life would just end?
- Are there times when the future looks hopeless?
- Do you ever feel like doing something drastic about your problems?

Examples of direct questions are:

- Do you ever feel like harming yourself?
- Have you ever deliberately harmed yourself?
- Do you ever feel suicidal?
- Do you sometimes feel like killing yourself?

There is no absolutely correct way of eliciting suicidal thoughts, and each doctor needs to establish his or her own method with which he or she feels comfortable. With some patients it may seem more appropriate to use only direct questions: each situation needs to be assessed on its own merits. Once it has been established that the patient does have suicidal thoughts, further questions need to be asked to assess their severity and the chances of the patient acting on them.

Questions used to explore further are:

- How frequent are these thoughts?
- How intense are they?
- Have you made any plans and are the means available?
- What has stopped you so far?
- How safe do you feel?

The patient can now be allowed ventilation of his or her feelings. It is important that the doctor shows interest and acknowledges the awfulness of how the patient feels. It is strange but true that the patients who feel that you understand how desperate they are do not have to prove it to you.

Parasuicide and its relationship to suicide

Parasuicide is a term that is virtually synonymous with attempted suicide, but which is intended to avoid the dispute over what are the actual intentions of those persons who take large overdoses but perhaps hope not to die. The relationship between suicide on the one hand and attempted suicide or parasuicide on the other, has been much studied by Hawton[66] and Morgan.[67] Substance abuse inpatients who have already harmed themselves are at particularly high risk for subsequent suicide in both the long and the short term. Parasuicide is commonest in the 15–25 year age group, with females far out-numbering males. Self-poisoning is the most frequently used method.

Facts about parasuicides:

- There are 100–300/100 000 population acts per year
- 25–30% are treated solely by their GP
- At least 20% repeat the act within the next 12 months
- 1–2% go on to complete suicide within the next 12 months
- 30% of people who commit suicide have self-harmed in the past

Assessment of suicide risk following an attempt

Not all people who deliberately self-harm kill themselves and predicting those who will is notoriously difficult. This does not mean that doctors should avoid making an in-depth risk assessment in every case. The following are guidelines for a *systematic* suicide risk assessment.

Prepare before seeing the patient

Look at the patient's past medical records if you have access to them and make sure that the patient is sufficiently conscious before the interview.

Establish rapport with the patient and take an accurate history

This will often involve interviewing other family members and friends. Attempt to understand the events leading up to the crisis and the *intent* behind the act. A full examination of the mental state should be carried out to establish any underlying psychiatric illness. With regard to *intent* it is important to establish the following:

- Was the act planned?

- Did the patient intend to die and did the patient think that the method was sufficient to cause death? The medical lethality of the method does not always correlate with the intent of the patient. Many patients believe that 10 temazepam tablets will kill them whereas 50 paracetamol will not.

- Were illegal drugs or alcohol involved?

- Did the patient leave a note?

- Did the patient make efforts to avoid being found?

- Did the patient self-harm in order to 'manipulate others'?

- Has the patient self-harmed previously and does he or she fall into any of the high-risk categories for suicide?

- Does the patient regret still being alive?

- Beware of the patient who denies suicidal intent but whose actions reveal a high risk (e.g. the patient left a note and went to great lengths not to be found).

The level of the patient's social support networks needs to be assessed. Once all the facts have been attained, the current suicide risk and the immediate risk of further self-harm can be established. Further management depends on this information.

Negotiate a management plan with the patient

If the current suicide risk is not great and the risk of further self-harm is minimal, hospital admission is not necessary and may in fact be counterproductive. However, it is always a reasonable course of action for a GP to refer a suicidal patient to a mental health care team for assessment. The specific treatment depends on the circumstances of the individual case. Medication, psychotherapy or referral to another agency may be appropriate. Before leaving the patient make sure that he or she has a real alternative to self-harm, such as a particular person to turn to, telephone numbers to ring, and so on. Arrange follow-up, either with yourself if appropriate, or with someone else. If the risk of suicide or further self-harm remains high, arrange admission to hospital, under compulsion if necessary. The patient may need to be admitted to a medical ward if there are medical complications. Remember that patients can be restrained under common law if they are in an immediate life-threatening situation.

Ending the interview

It was emphasized earlier that patients should be encouraged to talk about their suicidal feelings, their hopelessness and despair. This simple step uses such elementary communication techniques as saying 'tell me some more about that' or 'I was interested in what you were saying about ...'. Though the technique may be simple, the effect on the doctor may be trying. Even the most experienced physicians often still find it difficult to sit and hear the patient's undiluted despair and anguish.

One may be tempted to reassure such patients, for instance by telling them (what is likely to be true) that they will feel better about things in a few weeks' time. However, this reassurance is strongly contraindicated. The problem with it is that patients get the impression that you do not really understand how desperate their plight is, as otherwise you could not possibly be so smug about it. You run the risk of undoing all the good you have done in letting patients feel that you have been listening to them and really understanding how they feel.

Allowing patients to feel that you have heard what they are saying, that you really understand their despair, is the essential ingredient of the doctor's intervention here. You are using a well-known psychotherapeutic principle: that talking out problems avoids acting out problems. The doctor has to grit his or her teeth and let patients express their hopelessness without the comforting balm of reassurance.

How do you end such an interview? Sooner or later the doctor has to call a halt to the process of encouraging the patient to talk about his or her feelings. In fact, it is usually relatively easy to end this consultation. No dramatic answers to the patient's allegedly insoluble problems have to be put forward by the doctor. After giving the advice outlined above in 'Negotiate a management plan with the patient', basically you offer the patient another appointment. 'I should like to talk to you some more about this.' Usually the doctor and patient can agree on a sensible time at which to meet again. This prospect is enough to keep hope alive.

Prevention of suicide

The preventability of suicide has been widely debated within the medical profession. Some doctors believe that it is only by restricting the availability and the lethality of the methods available, such as adding methionine to paracetamol, that we will have an impact on the suicide rate.[68] Others believe that education programmes for GPs, particularly relating to treatment of depression, would be effective. One such programme was launched on the Swedish island of Gotland in 1983.[69] GPs were trained to recognize depression and treat it appropriately with antidepressants. This did indeed reduce the suicide rate. However, the effect was not maintained after the educational initiative was stopped. More recently, in the UK the Royal

College of Psychiatrists and the Royal College of General Practitioners have jointly launched the Defeat Depression Campaign to increase public awareness about depression and also to educate GPs and other health care professionals. It will be interesting to see if this does have an effect on the suicide rate. Meanwhile, GPs can employ the strategies mentioned above and their knowledge about suicide risk to help them make an accurate assessment in these often difficult situations.

The skills and training requirements of general practitioners in mental health today

Before considering how to improve recognition of depression in general practice, it is important to consider whether recognition actually results in patients getting better.

Recognition improves patient outcome

There is a little evidence that the act of aknowledging a person's depression has a slight therapeutic effect in itself (Freeling, personal communication), which makes intuitive sense. Helping someone to piece together their symptoms often helps, but treatment is then necessary to build upon this effect.

Patients recognized as having a psychiatric disorder by the GP are more likely to receive treatment and fare better in terms of psychopathology and social functioning than those whose depression is not recognized.[22,23] Initial severity, psychological reasons for encounter, recent onset, diagnostic category and psychiatric co-morbidity are all related to better recognition and outcome.[22,23]

How to improve recognition

An awareness of how GPs vary in their ability to recognize depression has led to a series of efforts to help GPs improve in this respect (Table 8). Such efforts include Balint training which consists of discussion in small peer groups of case reports, with an emphasis on acquiring an understanding of the patient rather than agreeing a diagnosis. The method relies on discussing the nature of the relationship and transaction between doctor and patient. Successful training does produce a significant change in a doctor's personality.[70] Originally, all groups were led by psychoanalysts; later, leadership spread to GPs who had themselves experienced the training. One issue often raised is the value of continuity of contact between the patient and the same GP, particularly during treatment of depression.

Education about the causes and effects of depression
   (a) medical students
   (b) vocational trainees ⎫ e.g. the Unit for Mental Health
   (c) established GPs   ⎭ Education in Primary Care
   (d) other primary health care professionals
   (e) the public (e.g. Defeat Depression Campaign)

Balint training

Increasing the continuity of care
   (a) personal lists
   (b) more/longer follow-up appointments

Training in interview skills (video feedback)

Screening questionnaires

Destigmatizing depression (Defeat Depression Campaign)

Table 8
Ways of improving the detection of depression

Questionnaires

Another question often asked is whether questionnaires can be used to replace the 'antennae' of the GP, or augment them. Screening by questionnaire does improve recognition, particularly in high-risk groups (e.g. postnatal women), but needs to be supplemented by the appropriate interview skills.[71] Many of the issues in improvement of recognition are educational, requiring the education of medical students, vocational trainees and GPs, and also public education of the general public to reduce stigma and encourage self-recognition, acknowledgement to the doctor and recognition by families.

Interviewing skills

Teaching interviewing skills to trainees can increase their accuracy in recognizing psychiatric disorders, although those who

Figure 3a
Poor interviewing technique

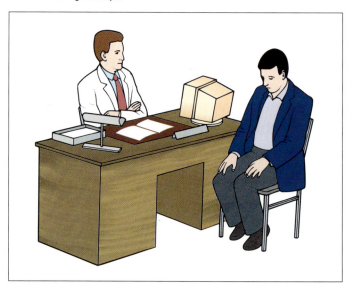

perform poorly at onset may also need instruction about approaches to management (Figure 3).[72,73]

The technique of problem-based interviewing[74] has successfully been taught to GP trainees[75] and established GPs.[76] The latter improved their skills in psychiatry, which were already good.[76] It is possible that the improvement in performance is related in part to the group work and not only to the technique learnt. Communication skills training of GPs increases patient satisfaction[77] and interviewing skills taught to undergraduates persist into professional life.[78] It is generally accepted that communication skills can be taught and that the subsequent benefits to medical practice are demonstrable, feasible on a routine basis and lasting.[79] When GPs are asked about their perceived training needs in mental health, communication skills and talking treatments are often at the top of their lists.[14]

Figure 3b
The most appropriate position for effective interviewing

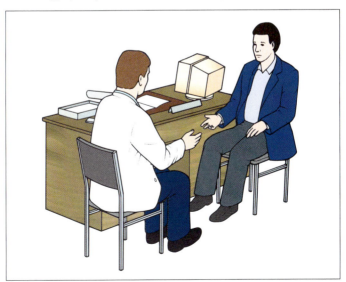

The Unit for Mental Health Education in Primary Care

The RCGP Senior Mental Health Education Fellowship was established in the UK in April 1992 with joint funding from the Department of Health, the Mental Health Foundation and the Gatsby Charitable Trust. The post was created to consider how to improve continuing medical education in mental health for GPs in England. The overall aim is to improve GP detection and management of mental illness, and this is being tackled with the assistance of the regional advisers in England, who have appointed several regional mental health education fellows. All but one of these fellows are GPs and they meet with the author (AT) residentially every 2 months to determine how best to support their GP tutors in running their continuing medical education (CME) programmes by providing educational materials in mental health and training on how to teach them. The educational materials cover depression, suicide, how to measure ability to identify psychiatric illness, problem-based interviewing, depression in the elderly, schizophrenia, depression in children and adolescents and alcohol misuse. It is the authors' wish that anyone who needs help in providing mental health education for GPs at a practice, a faculty, a post-graduate centre or a trainee group will contact their regional fellow or Dr André Tylee for help.

Summary

Table 9 provides the essential steps for GPs who wish to improve their ability to recognize depression. First, they need to remember that they are possibly missing depression in many of their patients who have concurrent physical illness and in consultations which do not start in a psychiatric mode. They may also miss depression by not asking many psychological questions. It is important to remain alert to the possibility of depression in all patients and to be willing to follow up any verbal or non-verbal cues wherever they appear in the consultation. Particular groups that should arouse a high level of suspicion include post-natal women, deaf, blind and dumb patients, the physically ill, elderly patients and alcoholics.

It is relatively easy to memorize and use the DSM-IV criteria or ICD-10 criteria for major depression. Knowledge of these criteria helps to achieve a more accurate diagnosis than only using, say, three or four favourite questions. It is important to

1 Have a high index of suspicion at all time especially when dealing with high risk groups, e.g.:

The physically ill

Patients with sensory impairment

Postnatal women

Elderly patients

Alcoholic patients

2 Memorize the diagnostic criteria (or have a convenient *aide memoire*)

3 Ask questions based on all the criteria whenever one is mentioned in the consultation

4 Review video recordings of your own consultations, preferably in a peer group

Table 9
Steps to improve recognition of depression

remember that one criterion (e.g. poor sleep) repeatedly reported still only counts as one of the nine criteria for major depression. Simply asking for the other eight criteria whenever one is mentioned should considerably increase the chance of recognizing an underlying major depression.

References

1   Thompson C, Affective disorders. In: Thompson C, ed., *The instruments of psychiatric research* (John Wiley and Sons Ltd: Chichester, 1989).

2   American Psychiatric Association, *Diagnostic and statistical manual of mental disorders,* 4th edn (American Psychiatric Association: Washington DC, 1994).

3   World Health Organisation, *ICD-10 classification of mental and behavioural disorders. Clinical descriptions and diagnostic guidelines* (WHO: Geneva, 1992).

4   Armstrong EA, Lloyd K, Management of depression in primary care (card produced for the Defeat Depression Campaign, Royal College of Psychiatrists, London).

5   Paykel ES, The background: extent and nature of the disorder. In: Herbst K, Paykel ES, eds, *Depression. An integrative approach* (Heinemann: Oxford, 1989).

6   Goldberg DP, Huxley P, *Mental illness in the community. The pathway to psychiatric care* (Tavistock: London, 1980).

7   Freeling P, Rao BM, Paykel ES et al, Unrecognized depression in general practice, *Br Med J* (1985) **290**:1880–3.

8   Bridges K, Goldberg D, Somatic presentation of depressive illness in primary care. In: Freeling P, Downey LJ, Malkin JC, eds, *The presentation of depression: current approaches* (The Royal College of General Practitioners: London, 1987).

9   Fahy TJ, Pathways of specialist referral of depressed patients from general practice, *Br J Psychiatry* (1974) **124**:231–9.

10 Blacker CVR, Clare AW, Depressive disorder in primary care, *Br J Psychiatry* (1987) **150**:735–51.

11 Sireling LI, Freeling P, Paykel ES et al, Depression in general practice: clinical features and comparison with out-patients, *Br J Psychiatry* (1985) **147**:119–25.

12 Sireling LI, Paykel ES, Freeling P et al, Depression in general practice: case thresholds and diagnosis, *Br J Psychiatry* (1985) **147**:113–19.

13 Marks JN, Goldberg D, Hillier VF, Determinants of the ability of general practitioners to detect psychiatric illness, *Psychol Med* (1979) **9**:337–53.

14 MORI Poll, conducted for Defeat Depression Campaign, London 1992.

15 MORI Poll, conducted for Defeat Depression Campaign, London 1995.

16 Bucholz KK, Robin LN, Who talks to a doctor about existing depressive illness? *J Affective Disord* (1987) **12**:241–250.

17 Bucholz KK, Dinwiddie SH, Influence of non-depressive symptoms on whether patients tell a doctor about depression, *Am J Psychiatry* (1989) **146**:640–44.

18 Blacker CVR, Clare AW, The prevalence and treatment of depression in general practice, *Psychopharmacology* (1988) **95**:S14–17.

19 Wright AF, A study of the presentation of somatic symptoms in general practice by patients with psychiatric disturbance, *Br J Gen Practice* (1990) **40**:459–63.

20 Mann AH, Jenkins R, Belsey E, The twelve month outcome of patients with neurotic illness in general practice, *Psychol Med* (1981) **11**:535–50.

21 Davenport S, Goldberg D, Millar T, How psychiatric disorders are missed during medical consultations, *Lancet* (1987) **ii**:439–40.

22 Ormel J, Koeter H, van den Brink W et al, The extent of non-recognition of mental health problems in primary care and its effect on management and outcome. In: Goldberg D, Tantam D, eds, *The public health impact of mental disorder* (Hogrefe-Huber: Basle, 1990) 154–64.

23 Ormel J, Van den Brink W, Koeter MWJ et al, Recognition, management and outcome of psychological disorders in primary care: a naturalistic follow-up study, *Psychol Med* (1990) **20**:909–23.

24 Tylee AT, Freeling P, Kerry S, Why do general practitioners recognize major depression in one woman patient yet miss it in another? *Br J Gen Practice* (1993) **43**:327–30.

25 Tylee A, Freeling P, The recognition, diagnosis and acknowledgement of depressive disorder by general practitioners. In: Herbst K, Paykel E, eds, *Depression: an integrative approach* (Heinemann: Oxford, 1989).

26 Schulberg HC, McClelland M, A conceptual model for educating primary care providers in the diagnosis and treatment of depression, *Gen Hosp Psychiatry* (1987) **9**:1–10.

27 Goldberg DP, Jenkins L, Millar T et al, The ability of trainee general practitioners to identify psychological distress among their patients, *Psychol Med* (1993) **23**:185–93.

28 Howie JGP, Porter AMD, Heaney DJ et al, Long to short consultation ratio: a proxy measure of quality of care for general practice, *Br J Gen Practice* (1991) **41**:48–54.

29 Truax CB, Carkhuff RR, *Toward effective counselling and psychotherapy: training and practice* (Aldine Atherton: Chicago, 1967).

30 Balwin DS, Priest RG, The Defeat Depression Campaign, *Primary Care Psychiatry* (1995) **1**:71–6.

31 Paykel ES, Priest RG, Recognition and management of depression in general practice: consensus statement, *Br Med J* (1992) **305**:1198–202.

32 Rutz W, Von Knorring L, Walinder J, Effect of an educational program for general practitioners on Gotland on the pattern of prescription of psychotropic drugs, *Acta Psychiat Scand* (1990) **82**:399–403.

33 Rutz W, Von Knorring L, Pihlgren H et al, An educational project on depression and its consequences: is the frequency of major depression among Swedish men under-rated, resulting in high suicidality? *Primary Care Psychiatry* (1995) **1**:59–63.

34 Frank E, Kupfer DJ, Peres JM et al, Three year outcome for maintenance therapies in recurrent depression, *Arch Gen Psychiatry* (1990) **47**:1093–99.

35 Kupfer DJ, Frank E, Peres JM et al, Five year outcome for maintenance therapies in recurrent depression, *Arch Gen Psychiatry* (1992) **49**:769–73.

36 Doogan DP, Caillard V, Sertraline in the prevention of depression, *Br J Psychiatry* (1992) **160**:217–22.

37 Montgomery SA, Dufou H, Brian S et al, The prophylactic efficacy of fluoxetine in unipolar depression, *Br J Psychiatry* (1988) **3**:69–76.

38 Montgomery SA, Dunbar GC, Paroxetine is better than placebo in relapse prevention and the prophylaxis of recurrent depression, Int Clin Psychopharmacol (1993) **8**:189–95.

39 Paykel ES, Hollyman JA, Freeling P et al, Predictors of therapeutic benefit from amitriptyline in mild depression: a general practice placebo controlled trial, *J Affective Disord* (1988) **14**:83–95.

40 Blashki TG, Mowbray R, Davies B, Controlled trial of amitriptyline in general practice, *Br Med J* (1971) **1**:133–8.

41 Thomson J, Rankin H, Ashcroft GW et al, The treatment of depression in general practice: a comparison of L-tryptophan, amitriptyline and a combination of L-tryptophan and amitriptyline with placebo, *Psychol Med* (1982) **12**:741–51.

42 Mynors-Wallis LM, Gath DH, Lloyd Thomas AR et al, Randomised clinical trial comparing problem solving treatment with amitriptyline and placebo for major depression in primary care, *Br Med J* (1995) **310**:441–5.

43 Thompson C, Thompson CM, The prescribing of antidepressants in general practice 2: a placebo-controlled trial of low-dose dothiepin, *Human Psychopharmacol* (1989) **4**:191–204.

44 Edwards JG, Selective serotonin reuptake inhibitors: a modest though welcome advance in the treatment of depression, *Br Med J* (1992) **304**:1644–6.

45 Hindmarch I, The psychopharmacological approach: effects of psychotropic drugs on car handling, *Int Clin Psychopharmacol* (1988) **3**:73–9.

46 Beck AT, Rush AJ, Shaw BF et al, *Cognitive therapy of depression: a treatment manual* (Guildford: New York, 1979).

47 Blackburn IM, Eunson KM, Bishop S, A two year naturalistic follow-up of depressed patients' treatment with cognitive therapy, pharmacotherapy and a combination of both, *J Affective Disord* (1986) **10**:67–75.

48 Klerman GL, Weissman MM, Rounsaville BJ et al, *Interpersonal psychotherapy of depression* (Basic books: New York, 1994).

49 Weissman MM, Prusoff BA, DiMascio A et al, The efficacy of drugs and psychotherapy in the treatment of acute depressive episodes, *Am J Psychiatry* (1979) **136**:555–8.

50 Weissman MM, Klerman GL, Prusoff BA et al, Depressed out-patients: results one year after treatment with drugs and/or interpersonal therapy, *Arch Gen Psychiatry* (1981) **38**:51–5.

51 Elkin I, Shea T, Watkins JT et al, National Institute of Mental Health treatment of depression collaborative research pro-gramme: general effectiveness of treatments, *Arch Gen Psychiatry* (1989) **46**:971–82.

52 Corney R, The effectiveness of attached social workers in the management of depressed female patients in general practice, *Psychol Med* (1984) **14** (Suppl 6): 47.

53 Corney RH, Marital problems and treatment outcome in depressed women, *Br J Psychiatry* (1987) **151**:652–9.

54 Holden JM, Sagovsky R, Cox JL, Counselling in general prac-tice settings: a controlled study of health visitor intervention in the treatment of post-natal depression, *Br Med J* (1989) **298**:223–6.

55 Secretary of State for Health, *The health of the nation: a strat-egy for health in England* (HMSO: London, 1992).

56 Secretary of State for Health, *Key area handbook: mental illness* (Department of Health: London, 1993).

57 Vassilas C, Morgan HG. General practitioners' contact with victims of suicide, *Br Med J* (1993) **307**:300–1.

58 Gunnell D, Recent studies of contacts with services prior to suicide: Somerset. In: Jenkins R, Griffiths S, Wylie I et al, eds, *The Prevention of Suicide* (HMSO: London, 1994) 114–20.

59 O'Donnell I, Farmer R, The limitations of official suicide statistics, *Br J Psychiatry* (1995) **166**:458–61.

60 Robins E, Murphy GE, Wilkinson RH et al, Some clinical considerations in the prevention of suicide based on a study of 134 successful suicides, *Am J Public Health* (1959) **49**:888–98.

61 Dorpat T, Ripley HS, A study of suicide in the Seattle area, *Comp Psychiatry* (1960) **1**:349–59.

62 Barraclough B, Bunch J, Nelson B et al, A hundred cases of suicide: clinical aspects, *Br J Psychiatry* (1974) **125**:355–73.

63 King E, Suicide in the mentally ill, An epidemiological sample and implications for six physicians, *Br J Psychiatry* (1994) **165**:658–63.

64 Cattell H, Jolly DJ, One hundred cases of suicide in elderly people, *Br J Psychiatry* (1995) **166**:451–7.

65 Hawton K, Assessment of suicide risk, *Br J Psychiatry* (1987) **150**:145–53.

66 Hawton K, Fagg J, Platt S et al, Factors associated with suicide after parasuicide in young people, *Br Med J* (1993) **306**:1641–4.

67 Morgan G, Long term risks after attempted suicide, *Br Med J* (1993) **306**:1626–7.

68 Gunnell D, Frankel S, Prevention of suicide: aspirations and evidence, *Br Med J* (1994) **308**:1227–33.

69 Rutz W, von Knorring L, Walinder J, Long term effects of an educational programme for general practitioners given by the Swedish Committee for the prevention and treatment of depression, *Acta Psychiatr Scand* (1992) **85**:83–8.

70 Balint M, Balint E, Gosling R et al, *A study of doctors* (Pitman Medical: London, 1965).

71 Hoeper EW, Nycz PD, Cleary PD et al, Estimated prevalence of RDC mental disorder in primary mental care, *Int J Mental Health* (1979) **8**:6–15.

72 Goldberg DP, Steele JJ, Smith C, Teaching psychiatric interviewing skills to family doctors, *Acta Psychiatr Scand* (1980) **62**:41–7.

73 Goldberg DP, Steele JJ, Smith C et al, Training family doctors to recognise psychiatric illness with increased accuracy, *Lancet* (1980) **ii**:521–3.

74 Lesser AL, Problem-based interviewing in general practice: a model, *Med Educ* (1985) **19**:209–304.

75 Gask L, Goldberg D, Lesser AL et al, Improving the psychiatric skills of the general practice trainee: an evaluation of a group training course, *Med Educ* (1988) **22**:132–8.

76 Gask L, McGrath G, Goldberg DP et al, Improving the psychiatric skills of established general practitioners: evaluation of group teaching, *Med Educ* (1987) **21**:362–8.

77 Evans J, Kiellerup FD, Stanley RO et al, A communication skills programme for increasing patients' satisfaction with general practice consultations, *Br J Med Psychol* (1987) **60**:373–8.

78 Maguire G, Fairbairn S, Fletcher C, Benefit of feedback training in interviewing as students persist, *Br Med J* (1986) **1**:268–70.

79 Simpson M, Buckman R, Stewart M et al, Doctor–patient communication: the Toronto Consensus Statement, *Br Med J* (1991) **303**:1385–7.

Index

A

Acute-phase treatment, 17
Addison's disease, 4
Affective disorder, 28
Age, and suicide risk, 27–8
Agitation, 1
Akathisia, 29
Alcoholism, 4, 23, 28–9
Amitriptyline, 23
Amphetamines, 4
Anaemia, 4
Antidepressants, 9, 15
Antipsychotic drugs, 20–1
Anxiety, 1, 20
Anxiolytics, 15
Appetite, loss of, 1
Attitudes, general practitioners, 12–13

B

Balint training, 39
Barbiturates, 4
Benzodiazepines, 4, 20–1
Bipolar affective disorder, 4, 21
Brain:
  carcinoma, 4
  disorders, 4
Brucellosis, 4
Bulimia, 20

C

Carcinoma, 4
Cerebrovascular accidents, 4

Clinical psychologists, 24
Cognitive behaviour therapy, 21–2
Communication skills, 41
Community psychiatric nurses (CPNs), 24
Continuation-phase treatment, 17
Corticosteroids, 4
Counselling, 21, 23
Cushing's syndrome, 4

D

Defeat Depression Campaign, 5, 9, 14, 15, 37
Dementia, 4
Department of Health, 42
Depression:
  criteria, 2–4, 5, 43
  definition, 1
  differential diagnosis, 4
  drug treatment, 15–21
  general practitioner skills and training, 38–44
  incidence, 6
  management of, 14–24
  non-drug treatment, 21
  patient features, 7, 9–11
  suicide, 25–37
  unacknowledged, 6–8, 11
Diagnosis, 4
Differential diagnosis, 4
Diuretics, 4
Drugs:
  antidepressants, 15
  differential diagnosis of depression, 4
  patient refusal of, 9
  suicide, 34

treatment of depression, 15–21
withdrawal symptoms, 4
DSM-IV criteria, 2, 43
Dysthymia, 3

K

Kidney disease, 4

E

Electroconvulsive therapy (ECT), 20
Endocrine conditions, 4
Epilepsy, 4
Eye-contact, general practitioners, 12

L

Lithium, 15, 20–1
Lofepramine, 18
Lung cancer, 4

F

Folate deficiency, 4

M

Major depression, 2–4
Manic-depressive disorder, 4
Mental Health Foundation, 42
Methionine, 36
Methyldopa, 4
Mianserin, 20
Moclobemide, 20
Monoamine oxidase inhibitors (MAOIs), 20
Mood changes, 1
Multiple sclerosis, 4
Muscarinic neurotransmitter systems, 20

G

Gatsby Charitable Trust, 42
General practitioners:
 assessment of suicide risk, 30–2, 33–6
 failure to acknowledge depression, 11–13
 skills and training, 38–44
Glandular fever, 4
Gotland, 14, 36

N

Neurosis, 28, 29
Neurotransmitter systems, 20
Noradrenergic neurotransmitter systems, 20

H

Haematological disorders, 4
Health of the Nation, 26
Hepatitis, 4
Herpes zoster, 4
Histaminergic neurotransmitter systems, 20
Hypnotics, 15
Hypothyroidism, 4

O

Obsessive–compulsive disorder, 23, 29
Overdoses:
 suicide, 34
 tricyclic antidepressants, 18

I

ICD-10 criteria, 4, 5, 43
Imipramine, 22
Incidence of depression, 6
Influenza, 4
International Classification of Diseases, 4
Interpersonal therapy, 22–3
Interviewing skills, 40–1
Iron deficiency anaemia, 4

P

Pancreatic carcinoma, 4
Panic attacks, 20, 29
Paracetamol, 34, 36
Parasuicide, 32–3
Parkinson's disease, 4
Personality disorders, 28, 29
Poisoning, parasuicide, 32
Prophylaxis, 17

Psychiatrists, 9, 23–4
Psychomotor retardation, 1, 19, 28
Psychotic depression, 20

Q

Questionnaires, 40

R

Renal failure, 4
Reserpine, 4
Reversible inhibitors of monoamine
    oxidase (RIMA), 20
Risk factors, suicide, 27–30
Rogerian counselling, 23
Royal College of General Practitioners,
    9, 14, 37
  Senior Mental Health Education
      Fellowship, 42
Royal College of Psychiatrists, 9, 14,
    36–7

S

Schizophrenia, 28, 29
Selective serotonin reuptake inhibitors
    (SSRIs), 19–20
  side-effects, 19
Senior Mental Health Education
    Fellowship, 42
Serotonin syndrome, 19
Side-effects:
  selective serotonin reuptake inhibitors
      (SSRIs), 19
  tricyclic antidepressants (TCAs), 18
Sleep, 1
Social workers, 24
Somatization, 7
'Subclinical' depression, 4
Substance abuse, 32
Suicide, 1, 25–37
  assessment of risk, 30–2,33–7
  Gotland educational programme, 14,
      36
  incidence, 25
  overdoses, 18
  parasuicide, 32–3
  prevention, 36–7
  risk factors, 27–30
Sweden, 14, 26, 36

T

Temazepam, 34
Thioridazine, 20
Trazodone, 20
Tricyclic antidepressants (TCAs),18
  side-effects, 18

U

Unemployment, and suicide risk, 27, 29

V

Venlafaxine, 20
Vitamin B_{12} deficiency, 4

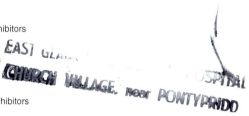